Skinny Like Me

5 - Day Detox Diet

Lose 5 Pounds in 5 Days

Recipes For Healthy Living

Shelby Daudlin

DEDICATION

To Sandra whom I love and thanks
for keeping me on the path

CONTENTS

Shelby Daudlin

Disclaimer

The opinions expressed in this book are published for educational and informational purposes only, and are not intended as a diagnosis, treatment or as a substitute for professional medical advice, diagnosis or treatment. Please consult a physician or other health care professional for your specific health care and/or medical needs or concerns. The information provided in this book is not intended to substitute for consultations with your doctor, nor medical advice specific to your health condition as we disclaim any liability arising from your use of the book or any adverse outcome of the information provided in this book for any reason, including but not limited to any misunderstanding or misinterpretation of the information provided here

Shelby Daudlin

1 - GOAL SETTING

OH NO!!

That's what most of say when we step on the scale for the first time in a long while. "The scale must be wrong" races through your mind, get on, get off, get on, get off, "nope it hasn't changed"!

What to do? Some of us at this point either choose to ignore the scale and carry on with life eating unhealthy, sitting on our buts in front of the television hoping to wake up one day to a fit and healthy body. For some of us this is a *wakeup call* to get off our butts and choose to lose weight and eat healthy. We all want a long life!

This book is designed to help you to do just that. Included is my 5 day Detox Diet, lose 5 pounds in 5 days. Included are home based exercises and lots of helpful information to get you on your way to and healthy new you. Anyone can do it right in your own home; all you need is a juice extractor and a blender.

First off we need to understand and evaluate your goals and what you would like to achieve. We will be using the S.M.A.R.T guide for achieving your goals as defined in this chapter.

Specific:

A specific goal has a much greater chance of being accomplished than a general goal. To set a specific goal you must ask yourself these questions:

*Who: Who is involved? Personal Trainer, etc

*What: What goals do I want to accomplish?

*Where: Identify a location, gym, etc

*When: Establish a time frame, date and time

*Which: Identify requirements and constraints, anything specific

*Why: Specific reasons, purpose of accomplishing the goal.

EXAMPLE: A general goal would be, "Get in shape." But a specific goal would say, "Following the steps in Skinny Like Me."

Measurable:

Establish concrete criteria for measuring progress toward the attainment of each goal you set.

When you measure your progress, you stay on track, reach your target dates, and experience the exhilaration of achievement that spurs you on to continued effort required to reach your goal.

Achievable:

When you identify goals that are most important to you, you begin to figure out ways you can make them come true. You develop the attitudes, abilities, skills, and financial capacity to reach them. You begin seeing previously overlooked opportunities to bring yourself closer to the achievement of your goals.

You can attain most any goal you set when you plan your steps wisely and establish a time frame that allows you to carry out those steps. Goals that may have seemed far away and out of reach eventually move closer and become attainable, not because your goals shrink, but because you grow and expand to match them. When you list your goals you build your self-image. You see yourself as worthy of these goals, and develop the traits and personality that allow you to possess them.

Realistic:

To be realistic, a goal must represent an objective toward which you are both *willing* and *able* to work. A goal can be both high and realistic; you are the only one who can decide just how high your goal should be. But be sure that every goal represents substantial progress.

A high goal is frequently easier to reach than a low one because a low goal exerts low motivational force. Some of the hardest jobs you ever accomplished actually seem easy simply because they were a labor of love.

Timely:

A goal should be grounded within a time frame. With no time frame tied to it there's no sense of urgency. If you want to lose 10 lbs, when do you want to lose it by? "Someday" won't work. But if you anchor it within a timeframe, "by May 1st", then you've set your unconscious mind into motion to begin working on the goal.
Your goal is probably realistic if you truly *believe* that it can be accomplished. Additional ways to know if your goal is realistic is to determine if you have accomplished anything similar in the past or ask yourself what conditions would have to exist to accomplish this goal.

The 10 Biggest Mistakes People Make in Setting Goals

1. There not written down. Unless a goal is written down, it is merely an aspiration lifeless and powerless. Once you commit it to writing, your setting your goals in motion. Clarify what you want and begin focusing on how to attain it.

2. Don't create too many. You need to stay focused on a manageable number of goals, too many and probably you won't reach any.

3. Don't set them for every aspect of your life focus on one area.

4. There not specific. Most goals even written ones suffer from being too vague. "I want to lose weight" or "I want to be fit" are too general.

5. There not measurable. The only way to know if you have achieved a goal is to measure it. "Lose 25 pounds" is much better than "lose weight." "Eat more vegetables" is better than "eat healthier" When in doubt, assign a number or a percentage.

6. They don't assign a due date. A deadline is one way to create urgency and force yourself to pay attention to what's important. Without a deadline, there's little pressure to get it done. It's easy to procrastinate.

7. They don't keep them visible. How many times have you written down a set of goals and never looked at them again? That's why you need a plan to keep them visible, whether that means reviewing them daily, weekly, or at some other regular interval.
8. They don't stretch out of their comfort zone. Safe goals are boring goals. Unless we set our goals outside our comfort zone, we won't find them compelling enough to actually follow through and achieve them. They shouldn't be unrealistic, but they should be challenging

9. They don't make them personally compelling. When you pursue a meaningful goal, it's exhilarating. Accomplishing it, even more so. This is why we need to write down a set of motivations for each goal identifying why it is important and what is at stake.
10. They don't identify the next action. You don't need an elaborate action plan for each goal. (Often this can just be a fancy way of procrastinating.) But you do need to identify the next action, so you can initiate and maintain momentum.
11.

2 – CHOOSING A JUICER

Why Juice?

There are many reasons to juice but I have three main reasons I believe why you should consider incorporating fresh juice, especially vegetable juice, into your lifestyle. Just remember the ratio is 80% vegetables to 20% fruit.

Fresh juice is the express way to health

1. Fresh juices go directly into your bloodstream and are therefore considered an express way to health. Unfortunately store bought juices contain virtually no nutrients due to the pasteurization process.

Offers a wide variety of fruit and vegetables to your diet

2. Many of us eat the same vegetables and fruits every day or, don't even eat them on a regular basis! With juicing, you can enjoy a wide variety of fruits and vegetables that you don't normally eat. Juicing is also the perfect way to consume the recommended daily serving of fruits and vegetables.

Fresh juice offers incredible health benefits

3. After regularly consuming freshly extracted fruit and vegetable juices, you will experience improved energy levels, digestion and mental clarity, clearer skin, and an overall sense of wellbeing.

Types of Juicers

So, you know three amazing health benefits of juicing and you're ready to get started. Now you're wondering what type of juicer is best for you.

There are many types of juicers available, varying in both quality and price. We will be looking at two main juicers on the market. A centrifugal juicer is a good start for beginners and is my choice for both quality and affordability.

Centrifugal Juicers

Centrifugal juicers are commonly available in retail outlets and are the cheapest type to purchase. These machines extract juice by pulverizing fruit and vegetables against a round cutting blade that spins very quickly against a stainless steel strainer. The centrifugal spinning motion of the cutting blade separates the juice from the pulp.

Cold Press / Masticating Juicers

These machines operate via a masticating (chewing) or cold press method to produce a superior juice to their centrifugal counterparts. In contrast to the rough extraction and high speeds of centrifugal juicers, cold press juicers operate at lower speeds and gently compress fruit and vegetables to 'squeeze' out their juice. While more costly, their slower and more thorough extraction rates produce a higher-quality juice, and more of it.

If you are looking for the **perfect** juicer and don't mind the cost, here is what to look for:

Ability to easily juice all greens, herbs and grasses (with a high yield)

Abel to juice fruits, including the soft varieties

Cold pressed, to produce a superior juice Low speed (rpm), to minimize oxidation and produce a longer lasting juice, able to make nut milks, easy to clean, low noise!

The best juicer on the market is the vertical cold-pressed masticating juicers.

My Recommendation

For the purposes and intent of this book I recommend the Breville Juice Fountain Plus, which is a Centrifugal juicer that really does the job and is priced for any budget.

This 850-watt professional juice extractor with a powerful 13,000 RPM motor juices both whole fruits and vegetables without the need for pre-chopping or pre-cutting. 2 speed electronic control juices soft and hard fruits in just five seconds. Patented 3" extra large centrifugal feed chute provides maximum juice extraction, and the two speed electronic control juices soft and hard fruits in just five seconds. Has a large, 2.5-liter capacity pulp container which is removable for easy cleaning and non-stop operation. Also includes a 1-liter juice pitcher with froth separator, instructions and recipes. Cord stores in base. All parts except motor housing are dishwasher safe.

BLENDERS

A good blender is a kitchen necessity, for making smoothies and for mixing non-juice able items into your juices.

TYPES OF BLENDERS

There are many types of blenders on the market but the best blender in my opinion to compliment the juice extractor is the NutriBullet. The NutriBullet easily blends and juices fruits and vegetables. All new Emulsifier blade busts opens seeds, cracks through stems, and shreds tough skin to access vital nutrients. Uses a 600 watt motor Includes a cookbook and pocket nutritionist Set includes hi-torque power base, 1 tall cup, 1 short cup, 1 short cup handled comfort lip ring, 1 handled short cup, 1 short cup comfort lip ring, extractor blade, milling blade, and stay-fresh re-sealable lids.

REGULAR BLENDERS

Regular blenders are good but leave behind pulp and do not blend seeds or nuts very well. But for our purposes a regular blender will do the trick.

3 – 5 Day Juice Detox Diet

THE PLAN

Wake up – 7:15am: 8 oz (250 ml) hot water with a lemon wedge

Breakfast – 8am: Yammy Sweet Potato Yum or Tropical Dream

Mid-Morning – 9:30am: Drink 16 oz of Coconut Water* or electrolyte based drink

Lunch – 11am: Good Greens or Green Time

Afternoon snack – 2pm: Blood Transfusion or Afternoon Delight

Dinner – 5pm: Green Jeans or Cilantro of the Lambs

Evening – 8pm: Summer Breeze or Purple Haze

Bedtime – 9pm: Drink herbal tea – Your Choice

Throughout the day: Drink lots of water

*Drink One Juice at Meal Time Alternating Daily.

*I recommend preparing the juices according to the Gram Weight for best results

* The Percent Daily Values are based on a 2,000 calorie diet, so your values may change depending on your calorie needs. The values here may not be 100% accurate because the recipes have not been professionally evaluated nor have they been evaluated by the U.S. FDA. All nutrient values are calculated from the USDA nutrition database

What's the Detox Diet?

A commitment to drinking and eating fresh fruits and vegetables for a period of time in order to lose weight or stimulate your metabolism. Start healthy habits that stimulate your body and get your body back in track for optimal wellness. The 5-Day Detox Diet involves drinking only fresh juice for 5 days.

Why Detox?

The Detox Diet is the perfect way to stimulate your system with fresh, clean foods. When you consume fruits and vegetables, your system is flooded with an abundance of vitamins; minerals that help your body become strong, look beautiful and help fight diseases.

Why Will The 5-Day Detox Diet Help?

• Stimulate your system
• Promote weight loss
• Strengthen your immune system
• Promote clearer skin
• Detoxify your internal organs such as your Liver, Kidneys
• Promote a healthy digestion system and cleanse your intestines

Who Can Detox?

Detoxing can be done by everyone with a few exceptions. Please don't attempt a Detox if you are pregnant or nursing, under 18 or have a severe medical condition. Check with your doctor before starting any Detox program.

Calorie Counting:

Our 5-Day Detox Diet is designed to provide approximately 1,262 maximum calories or less per day. It's a good idea to keep track of your daily caloric intake. Drinking vegetable juice and water will aid in your weight loss.

Expectations:

In the beginning, you may experience some setbacks. Don't worry that's all part of the detox process. As you start this 5-Day Detox you will be eliminating all solid foods, so you may experience some emotional distress along with some physical symptoms. Be prepared to be strong.

Ready to Detox:

The cleaner you eat the better the Detox Diet will work and the faster you will lose weight. A week or so before you start your Detox remove all processed meats, fast foods, white flours, sugar, desserts, dairy and fried food, especially alcohol and caffeine from your diet. Stay hydrated at *least* 8 cups per day, or more. Get lots of sleep. Eat more salads and vegetables and drink at least one fresh juice per day from the recipes provided.

Medication:

Continue to take your non-prescription vitamins and supplements during the Detox Diet and continue with your regular prescribed medications.

Exercise:

Exercise is important during your Detox, but reduce the intensity. You'll want to take it easy as you maybe experiencing light headedness and fatigue. You will be eating fewer calories and proteins as well as carbohydrates than usual. So adjust your workout accordingly. It's crucial to maintain your hydration during the detox, so be sure to drink plenty of fluids during your workout including electrolyte rich fluids. Walking, yoga, cycling are good activities to do during your Detox.

Possible Side Effects or Symptoms:

Beyond the benefits eating healthier, there are other potentially serious side effects of a detox that you need to be aware of. If any of these symptoms occur please consult your physician. Most side effects are temporary and will include but are not limited to: fatigue, headache, dizziness, low blood sugar, constipation and diarrhea. Adjustments to your Detox plan like increasing your fluid intake by drinking more electrolyte water and these side effects can often be resolved within the first few days.

If you are in any way concerned, contact your doctor immediately. If you experience any of the following symptoms, please stop the Detox and contact your physician: fainting, extreme dizziness, low blood pressure, significant weight loss, vomiting and severe diarrhea.

After you're Detox:

The Detox Diet doesn't stop after 5 days. Going forward, you can keep juicing by including a juice or two a day and incorporate more fruits and vegetables into your diet. If you have insignificant weight loss within the 5 days, you can restart the Detox Diet for another 5 day period. The first 3 days of any detox are typically the hardest.

Seeds & Berries – Natures Super Food

Seeds and berries are a very important part of the detox process they add lots of nutritional benefits.

CHIA: Balance Blood Sugar, add healthy omega-3 oil to your diet, Feel more energized all day long, Add age-defying anti-oxidants, and cut cravings for food.

ACAI: Appetite suppression mechanisms that aid individuals who need weight loss, Improved digestive capacities, Aids in the detoxification of the body through its high fiber content, May improve the overall appearance of the skin, due to high antioxidant qualities, May aid in improved heart health, May aid to reduce cholesterol levels, May aid in the prevention of cancer, heart disease, and stroke, May aid in reducing loose stools and diarrhea, May reduce the incidence of allergies.

GOJI: Some studies using goji berry juice found possible benefits in mental well-being and calmness, athletic performance, happiness, quality of sleep, and feelings of good health.

WHEATGRASS: Wheatgrass contains up to 70% chlorophyll, chlorophyll washes drug deposits from the body, Chlorophyll neutralizes toxins in the body, Chlorophyll helps purify the liver, Chlorophyll improves blood sugar problems, and Wheatgrass is a superior detoxification agent. Wheatgrass is also high in iron, magnesium, calcium, selenium, amino acids, and vitamins A, E, C, K and B-complex.

HEMP HEARTS: Raw hemp provides a broad spectrum of health benefits, including: weight loss, increased and sustained energy, rapid recovery from disease or injury, lowered cholesterol and blood pressure, reduced inflammation, improvement in circulation and immune system as well as natural blood sugar control.

FLAXSEED: Some call it one of the most powerful plant foods on the planet. There's some evidence it may help reduce your risk of heart disease, cancer, stroke, and diabetes. That's quite a tall order for a tiny seed that's been around for centuries. Omega-3 essential fatty acids, "good" fats that have been shown to have heart-healthy effects. Each tablespoon of ground flaxseed contains about 1.8 grams of plant omega-3s. Lignans, which have both, plant estrogen and antioxidant qualities. Flaxseed contains 75 to 800 times more lignans than other plant foods. Fiber, Flaxseed contains both the soluble and insoluble types.

To use these super food seeds make you juice as usual and add the recommended amount of seeds in your blender add your juice and blend for about sixty seconds and enjoy. You should add one type of seed to each juice at mealtimes.

MACA: is another incredible food you can add into your juices. The maca root is a superfood from Peru, helping the body adapt to environmental stress. Maca is wild harvested and consumed as a medicinal plant. The Inca warriors used maca to increase their strength and energy. It is also a powerful aphrodisiac and balances hormones, as with all stimulants, a little goes along way, so I recommend moderation.

Digestion

PROBIOTICS: Probiotics are increasingly being used and evaluated to help with digestive health. However, probiotic benefits are strain specific and thus different probiotics may have unique benefits. Your body needs beneficial bacteria for a number of things. But these bacteria are fragile. Common issues such as diet, changes in routine, travel, and stress can disrupt your natural healthy intestinal flora. Health benefits: Relieves and manages the symptoms of Irritable Bowel Syndrome (IBS)

Benefits Juicing May Help With

Lower Cholesterol

Digestion

Bone Protection

Lung Cancer Prevention

Breast Cancer Prevention

Alzheimer's Prevention

Colon Cancer Prevention

Liver Cancer Prevention

Macular Degeneration Prevention

Improved Complexion

Improving Eyesight

Reduce Water Retention

Stroke Prevention

Reduce Inflammation

Increased Blood Circulation

Blood Cleanse

Cancer Prevention

Immune System

Lower Blood Pressure

Weight Loss

Heart Disease Prevention

Increased Libido

Shelby Daudlin

Health Conditions

These are some health condition juicing could help with

Acidosis	Fatigue	Osteoporosis
Acne	Fever	Ovarian Cancer
Allergies	Flu	Pain
Alzheimer's Disease	Gall Bladder Stones	Poor Memory
Anemia	Hangover	Prostate Cancer
Anxiety	Headache	Rheumatism
Arthritis	High Blood Pressure	Muscle Spasms
Asthma	High Cholesterol	Nausea
Bladder Cancer	Indigestion	Sinus Congestion
Bloating	Itching	Skin Cancer
Breast Cancer	Kidney Stones	Stomach Cancer
Cancer	Leukemia	Stress
Cervical Cancer	Liver Disease	Stroke
Cold	Lung Cancer	Low Libido
Constipation	Menstrual Cycle	Colon Cancer

Shelby Daudlin

Breakfast Juice
Yammy Sweet Potato Yum

Ingredients – Makes One Serving – 15oz

Apple - 1 medium (3" dia) 182g

Orange (peeled) - 1 large (3-1/16" dia) - 184g

Pears – 1 Large - 230g

Sweet Potato - 1 - 5" long – 130g

Celery – 1 stalk, large - 64g

Dash of cinnamon on top

Directions

Process all ingredients in a juicer, shake or stir add ice and serve in 20oz glass.

*Add one super food seed daily (optional) – Blend with juice in a blender

ACAI add 15Cal/Tbsp – GOJI add 100Cal/.25 cup – HEMP add 170Cal/ 3 Tbsp – CHIA add 60Cal/Tbsp – WHEATGRASS add 35Cal/8 grams

Nutrition per serving:
251Cal; 3.8g protein; 76mg carbohydrates;
.72g fat; 012g saturated fat; 2.1g fiber; 45g sugar; 89mg salt

Breakfast Juice
Tropical Dream

Ingredients – Makes One Serving – 15oz

Mango - 1 - 336g

Orange - 1 large (3-1/16" dia) - 184g

Pineapple - 1 cup - 165g

Kale - 4 leaf - 140g

Ginger Root – 0.58 thumb (1" dia) – 14g

Directions

Process all ingredients in a juicer, shake or stir add ice and serve in 20oz glass.

*Add one super food seed daily (optional) – Blend with juice in a blender

ACAI add 15Cal/Tbsp – GOJI add 100Cal/.25 cup – HEMP add 170Cal/ 3 Tbsp – CHIA add 60Cal/Tbsp – WHEATGRASS add 35Cal/8 grams

Nutrition per serving:
332Cal; 8g protein; 84mg carbohydrates;
3g fat; .44g saturated fat; 1g fiber; 56g sugar; 79mg salt

Shelby Daudlin

Lunch Juice
Good Greens

Ingredients – Makes One Serving – 15oz

Apples - 1 medium (3" dia) - 182g

Celery - 2 stalk, large (11"-12" long) - 128g

Cucumber - 1 cucumber (8-1/4") - 301g

Kale - 4 leafs with stems (8-12") - 140g

Ginger Root – 0.58 thumb (1" dia) - 14g

Lemon - 1 wedge or slice (1/8 of one 2-1/8" dia) - 7g

Directions

Process all ingredients in a juicer, shake or stir add ice and serve in 20oz glass.

*Add one super food seed daily (optional) – Blend with juice in a blender

ACAI add 15Cal/Tbsp – GOJI add 100Cal/.25 cup – HEMP add 170Cal/ 3 Tbsp – CHIA add 60Cal/Tbsp – WHEATGRASS add 35Cal/8 grams

Nutrition per serving:
148Cal; 15g protein; 38mg carbohydrates;
1.6g fat; .26g saturated fat; .8g fiber; 18g sugar; 116mg salt

Lunch Juice
Green Times

Ingredients – Makes One Serving – 15oz

Apples - 1 medium (3" dia) - 182g

Celery - 2 stalk, large (11"-12" long) - 128g

Parsley - 1 handful - 40g

Spinach – 2 handfuls - 50g

Cucumber - 1 cucumber (8-1/4") - 301g

Ginger Root – 0.58 thumb (1" dia) - 13g

Lime (with rind) - 1 fruit (2" dia) - 67g

Directions

Process all ingredients in a juicer, shake or stir add ice and serve in 20oz glass.

*Add one super food seed daily (optional) – Blend with juice in a blender

ACAI add 15Cal/Tbsp – GOJI add 100Cal/.25 cup – HEMP add 170Cal/ 3 Tbsp – CHIA add 60Cal/Tbsp – WHEATGRASS add 35Cal/8 grams

Nutrition per serving:
116Cal; 13g protein; 35mg carbohydrates;
1g fat; 023g saturated fat; 1.2g fiber; 19g sugar; 122mg salt

Shelby Daudlin

Afternoon Juice
Blood Transfusion

Ingredients – Makes One Serving – 15oz

Bosc Pear - 1 small - 148g

Beet Root - 1 beets (3" dia) - 175g

Carrots - 1 large (7-1/4" to 8-/1/2" long) - 72g

Celery – 2 stalk, large (11"-12" long) - 128g

Cucumber - 1 cucumber (8-1/4") - 301g

Ginger Root – 1/2 thumb - 12g

Directions

Process all ingredients in a juicer, shake or stir add ice and serve in 20oz glass.

*Add one super food seed daily (optional) – Blend with juice in a blender

ACAI add 15Cal/Tbsp – GOJI add 100Cal/.25 cup – HEMP add 170Cal/ 3 Tbsp – CHIA add 60Cal/Tbsp – WHEATGRASS add 35Cal/8 grams

Nutrition per serving:
147Cal; 5g protein; 44mg carbohydrates;
.92g fat; .207g saturated fat; 1.5g fiber; 26g sugar; 208mg salt

Afternoon Juice
Afternoon Delight

Ingredients – Makes One Serving – 15oz

Apples - 3 medium (3" dia) - 224g

Carrots - 3 large (7-1/4" to 8-/1/2" long) - 216g

Ginger Root – 1/2 thumb - 12g

Directions

Peel Mango and process all ingredients in a juicer, shake or stir add ice and serve in a 20oz glass.

*Add one super food seed daily (optional) – Blend with juice in a blender

ACAI add 15Cal/Tbsp – GOJI add 100Cal/.25 cup – HEMP add 170Cal/ 3 Tbsp – CHIA add 60Cal/Tbsp – WHEATGRASS add 35Cal/8 grams

Nutrition per serving:
219Cal; 2.5g protein; 68mg carbohydrates;
1g fat; .18g saturated fat; 2g fiber; 109g sugar; 9mg salt

Dinner Juice

Green Jeans

Ingredients – Makes One Serving – 15oz

Apples - 1 medium (3" dia) - 546g

Orange (peeled) - 1 large (3-1/16" dia) - 184g

Celery - 2 stalk, large (11"-12" long) - 256g

Spinach - 5 handful - 125g

Ginger Root – ½" thumb - 8g

Lemon (with rind) - 1 wedge or slice (1/8 of one 2-1/8" dia lemon) - 7g

Directions

Peel the orange. Process all ingredients in a juicer, shake or stir add ice and serve in 20oz glass.

*Add one super food seed daily (optional) – Blend with juice in a blender

ACAI add 15Cal/Tbsp – GOJI add 100Cal/.25 cup – HEMP add 170Cal/ 3 Tbsp – CHIA add 60Cal/Tbsp – WHEATGRASS add 35Cal/8 grams

Nutrition per serving:
134Cal; 4.8g protein; 40mg carbohydrates;
.94g fat; .16g saturated fat; 1.4g fiber; 27g sugar; 143mg salt

Dinner Juice
Cilantro of the Lambs

Ingredients – Makes One Serving – 15oz

Apple - 1 medium (3" dia) - 182g

Carrots - large (7-1/4" to 8-/1/2" long) - 72g

Cilantro - 1 handful - 34g

Collard Greens - 1 handful - 36g

Kale - 4 leafs -140g

Pepper (sweet red) - medium (approx 2-3/4" long, 2-1/2 dia.) - 119g

Directions

Process all ingredients in a juicer, shake or stir add ice and serve in 20oz glass.

*Add one super food seed daily (optional) – Blend with juice in a blender

ACAI add 15Cal/Tbsp – GOJI add 100Cal/.25 cup – HEMP add 170Cal/ 3 Tbsp – CHIA add 60Cal/Tbsp – WHEATGRASS add 35Cal/8 grams

Nutrition per serving:
146Cal; 7g protein; 38mg carbohydrates;
1.7g fat; .18g saturated fat; 1.1g fiber; 19g sugar; 92mg salt

Shelby Daudlin

Evening Juice

Summer Breeze

Ingredients – Makes One Serving – 15oz

Apples - 2 medium (3" dia) - 364g

Carrots - 7 medium - 427g

Oranges (peeled) - 2 small (2-3/8" dia) - 192g

Directions

Process all ingredients in a juicer, shake or stir add ice and serve in 20oz glass.

*Add one super food seed daily (optional) – Blend with juice in a blender

ACAI add 15Cal/Tbsp – GOJI add 100Cal/.25 cup – HEMP add 170Cal/ 3 Tbsp – CHIA add 60Cal/Tbsp – WHEATGRASS add 35Cal/8 grams

Nutrition per serving:
199Cal; 4.3g protein; 62mg carbohydrates;
1.1g fat; .16g saturated fat; 2.1g fiber; 39g sugar; 208mg salt

Evening Juice

Purple Haze

Ingredients – Makes One Serving – 15oz

Apple - 1 medium (3" dia) - 182g

Beet Root - 1 beet - (3" die) - 175g

Celery - 2 stalk, medium (7-1/2" - 8" long) - 80g

Cider Vinegar (apple) - 1 tbsp - 5g

Ginger Root – 0.58 thumb (1" dia) – 15g

Grapes - 10 grape - 60g

Lemon (with peel) - 1 wedge or slice (1/8 of one 2-1/8" dia lemon) - 7g

Directions

The apple cider vinegar is optional. Process all ingredients in a juicer, shake or stir add ice and serve in a 20oz glass.

*Add one super food seed daily (optional) – Blend with juice in a blender

ACAI add 15Cal/Tbsp – GOJI add 100Cal/.25 cup – HEMP add 170Cal/ 3 Tbsp – CHIA add 60Cal/Tbsp – WHEATGRASS add 35Cal/8 grams

Nutrition per serving:
121Cal; 3.08g protein; 37mg carbohydrates;
.73g fat; .09g saturated fat; 1.3g fiber; 22g sugar; 142mg salt

4 – HOME EXERCISES

Workout for: Men, Women and Children

Body parts: Full body workout

Equipment: No equipment required

The Workout

This is a 20 minute home workout routine is perfect for the busy person on the go who doesn't have time to run out to the gym daily. In just 20 short minutes, you will work every single muscle in your body, accelerate your metabolism so you can burn fat faster, and improve your cardiovascular fitness. Do this at least three times per week and it's all you need to start looking and feeling great!

Workout instructions

For best results, begin with a five minute light cardio workout. Skipping rope, jogging on the spot, or even marching on the spot.

This routine consists of a circuit workout, alternating between strength based exercises along with cardio focused movements and core exercises to firm up your stomach.

Perform one exercise after the next only resting for as long as you have to in order to put forth a good effort with each exercise you do.

Aim to complete 15 reps of each exercise and then once the entire circuit is complete, rest for 2 minutes and repeat one more time through. Be sure that you always maintain good form to prevent injury and see the best possible results.

Strength based exercises: Pushups, Squats, Planks, Superman, Bridge

Cardio focused movements: Jumping Jacks, Burpees, Mountain Climbers, Bicycle Crunches

Core exercises: Bicycle Crunches, Dive Bombers, Cross Body Crunch, Jackknife Crunches, Weighted Twist

You can find lots of examples of these exercises on the Internet.

A good web site for body weight exercises is

www.workoutlabs.com

References

* Pages 3 – 5 Goal Setting: http://en.wikipedia.org/wiki/Goal_setting

*Page 7 & 8 – The 10 Biggest Mistakes People Make in Setting Goals: Michael Hyatt, former Chairman and CEO of Thomas Nelson Publishers

*Page 11 – Coconut Water as an electrolyte base drink: http://healthandwellness.kaplan.edu/articles/nutrition/Coconut%20water%20-%20Is%20it%20really%20natures%20sport%20drink.html

*Pages 15 & 16 Seeds & Berries: http://green-mom.com/topics/nutrition/why_are_superfoods_so_super.html#.U0vIglVdWSo

*Pages 17 & 28 – Health Benefits, Nutritional Facts and Recipes Ideas: http://juicerecipes.com

ABOUT THE AUTHOR

Shelby Daudlin has been in the Health and Fitness industry since 2008. Shelby is a Personal Trainer Specialist certified in Resist-A-Ball, Free Weights and Nutrition. He has taught Boot Camps as well as private in home Personal Training.

Shelby has had many successful clients meet their goals and maintain healthy lives. Shelby wrote this book to help people reach their personal goals and become healthy and confident.

We hope you enjoy this book and it helps you reach all your goals.